DOCTOR-TO-DOCTOR: AVOIDING FINANCIAL SUICIDE

Gary D. Steinman
MD, PhD

WITH TECHNICAL ASSISTANCE FROM
ALAN R. POLLACK, ESQ
AND
DAVID L. SCHWARTZ, CPA

Baffin Books, Inc.
New York, NY
1998

DOCTOR-TO-DOCTOR: AVOIDING FINANCIAL SUICIDE

By Gary D. Steinman

Published by:
  Baffin Books, Inc
  4601 Broadway
  Astoria, New York 11103 U.S.A.
     E-mail: BAFFINBOOKS@JUNO.COM

All rights reserved. No part of this book may be reproduced or transmitted in any form or by any means, electronic or mechanical, including photocopying, recording or by any information storage and retrieval system without written permission from the author, except for the inclusion of brief quotations in a review.

Copyright © 1998 by Gary D. Steinman
First printing - 1998
Printed by: Patterson Printing
Printed in the United States
Cover design: Boccio Design Group

   Publisher's Cataloging-in-Publication
      (Provided by Quality Books, Inc)

Steinman, Gary D.
  Doctor-to-doctor : avoiding financial suicide / Gary D. Steinman ; with technical assistance from Alan R. Pollack and David L. Schwartz. -- 1st ed.
    p. cm.
    Includes index.
    Preassigned LCCN:98-71744
    ISBN: 0-9665105-0-X

     1.Medicine--Practice. 2.Physicians--
         Finance, Personal.
  I. Title.

  R728.S84 1998   610',681
                         QBI98-791

DEDICATION

This book is written in honor of my mother,

Mildred Steinman, LPN

who sensitized me to the benevolence of medical practice, and my father,

Morris Steinman, MD*
(*Metals Dealer)

who introduced me to the fundamentals of good, ethical business practices.

ז"ל

בס"ד

"Take heed and care diligently for your lives."

Deuteronomy 4:9

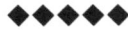

"God helps them that help themselves."

"There are three faithful friends - an old wife, an old dog, and ready money."

"When the well's dry, we know the worth of water."

"Little strokes fell great oaks."

"A word to the wise is enough."

"Remember that time is money."

Benjamin Franklin

INTRODUCTION

In much the same way that a well-trained physician actively manages the medical problem of a patient under his[1] care, so too should he be prepared to manage his own financial and economic health. Just as he must prudently select consultants to assist in the resolution of a medical problem, so too should he wisely choose financial advisers to provide applicable opinions and suggestions. In the end it is the physician himself who must elect the final approach to take, and be prepared to modify that approach depending on how events unfold.

---

[1] The generic terms "he" and "his" should be taken to refer equally to female physicians throughout this book.

The student doctor[2] must absorb an immense volume of material to prepare himself for independent clinical work. As a result, unfortunately, he is typically unenlightened to the special knowledge needed to effectively control and direct his own financial future. Most new physicians (and many seasoned practitioners, for that matter) do not have a clue about issues related to disciplined spending, effective business practices, and wise investing in the real world, following residency. For philosophical reasons, doctors may feel that attention to monetary issues taints their dedication to helping people, until the accounts payable start coming due. The

---

[2] The terms "doctor" and "physician" used in this text embrace <u>all</u> health care providers including dentists, osteopaths, optometrists, podiatrists, MD's, physical therapists, veterinarians, nurse practitioners, chiropractors, psychologists, etc.

converse is in fact true, namely, that a well-run office can better serve the community of patients seeking health care services there.

The managed care revolution has diminished the income expectations of the health care provider. However, the professional who has struggled through medical training for the purpose of aiding people is no less a dedicated, ethical, and effective physician if his financial life is properly arranged and in order. A doctor is entitled to be compensated for his time and expertise, just as the merchant should be paid for the computer he sells him to run his practice.

With the prestige and money which medical practice imparts, the typical doctor is mesmerized by the expectation that he may attain wealth in excess of $1,000,000 during his career. However, because of disregard and indifference, in his early professional years he might not prepare for the needs of later years. Funds are consumed with luxuries; accounts receivable are ignored too easily because of ineffective bookkeeping. Essential instruments which should be implemented early on, to set the stage for immediate and future financial security for himself and his dependents, are not initiated. These include life insurance, children's educational savings, and pension, among others. They are put off to a later date when it may, in fact, leave insufficient time for adequate accumulation and effective protection.

Doctors are prime targets for lenders who are anxious to extend credit to professionals with the acknowledged potential for strong future earnings. For the young practitioner it is an overwhelming temptation to "buy now and pay later," with new debt added on to outstanding educational loans. In this way, much of his career is a struggle to meet repayment demands and postpone more important issues, such as pension and savings "for a rainy day." Many doctors reach their 50's and begin to consider slowing down or even retiring, only to find that they must continue working hard for several more years just to "make ends meet." Many very successful practices are tragically reduced to bankruptcy because of inadequate planning.

This book presents an introduction to key concepts and terms which are vital for the doctor to understand, so that he may map out an appropriate strategy from day #1. It will also give him insight so that germane questions can be posed to financial advisers. However, only the individual himself can truly care enough about his own professional, financial, and personal life to maximize reasonable earnings. He must not delegate to others the responsibility for making major decisions because of the fear of a mistake or the assumption that he does not know (or care to know) enough about the subject to act wisely, effectively, and independently.

Most conscientious advisers, lawyers, business managers, insurance agents, and accountants endeavor to help the doctor satisfy his financial needs through the application of their knowhow from their perspective. However, in the end, it is the doctor alone who must decide if any particular advice is really in his best interest. He should not rely on the trite adage health care providers traditionally used with their patients:"Trust me, I know what is best for you." The patient population today is more aware and now demands informed disclosures. Likewise, the doctor <u>must</u> comprehend all details of the plans being proposed for his financial health before he consents to them. He must take command and be on top of all activities within and outside his office, without relinquishing the authority over key decisions and functions to others.

Contrary to popular belief among doctors, physicians are not all-knowing in every field of human endeavor nor do they have unlimited earning potential. Managed care has jumped in when it became apparent that money available for medical care is not limitless. Similarly, the physician needs to understand that his money is not unlimited. He must learn how to administer his expenditures knowledgeably and insightfully.

In the early years of practice, he may have to forgo the big car, the big house, and the big vacation, even if lenders are willing to provide the capital to meet these dreams. It is the long term that must be at the forefront of every doctor's game plan. Doctors do not "deserve" these treats any more than any other working person, until they are able to methodically resolve the more critical issues first. A car will only travel as far as the gasoline put into it will allow. Similarly, each person should limit his present spending to his currently available cash, and funds he can reasonably expect to have accessible, without sacrificing safety and security in the near or long term. This requires discipline, self-control, and maturity.

Sensible planning should mean a slow, steady, lifelong growth of net worth, rather than a fling at making a quick killing with high risk investments. This approach results in a gradual rise in one's standard of living, rather than an abrupt change which acutely swells debt obligations.

Deficit spending may be standard operating procedure for governments but can be disastrous for individuals.

For some people it is difficult to contemplate their own mortality or potential for disability, especially during the youthful, healthy years. Young doctors think that only their patients get sick. However, doctors are real people too, and they must confront the possibility of these needs arising earlier than they may have hoped for or anticipated. Thus, early planning is vital. Family security is at stake.

This book is written with the assumption that the doctor will enter solo practice. Therefore, little is specifically directed to negotiating contracts with groups. However, the same principles that are intended here for the individual apply equally to members of group practices.

From the inception of a practice, attention must be given to funds needed to cover equipment, salaries, insurance, and rent. A modest beginning can be embellished as income grows.

The subjects that follow are alphabetized for convenient access. They were carefully selected by and from the perspective of a practicing physician to be among those about which every doctor should have a working knowledge and understanding. This book is designed as a handy reference for initial orientation into areas of particular interest to the practitioner. It is not intended to be an encyclopedic source of information. Each subject is condensed to one page and is presented as an introduction to the salient features of a fundamental definition, concept, or function. Subjects are cross-referenced for continuity. In the same way that physicians update their professional skills through their continuing medical education, the doctor/spouse/parent must continue to sharpen his knowledge in the economic realm throughout life to effectively serve his key functions within the personal sphere as well.

SPECIAL NOTICE

In no way is this book intended to function as an exhaustive, detailed legal reference or primary source. Before making vital financial decisions, the reader must consult with proper experts and authoritative sources for more complete, definitive explanations and advice as needed. This book is designed to provide an introductory overview of applicable information in the subject matter covered. It is sold with the understanding that the author and the publisher are not engaged in the profession of rendering legal, accounting, investment, insurance, or other financial services.

Every effort has been devoted to make this book as thorough, concise, and accurate as possible. Errors related to typographical and technical matters may have entered the manuscript unintentionally. The most up-to-date legal rulings, legislation, and opinions should be obtained from appropriate professional experts. This educational text should only be used as a general guide and not as an ultimate source for making financial decisions.

Therefore, the author, consultants, and publisher of this book shall have neither liability nor responsibility to any person or entity with respect to any loss or damage caused, or alleged to be caused, directly or indirectly, by the information contained in the book. If you do not wish to be bound by these limitations and precautions, you may return this book in resalable condition to the publisher or his distributor for a full refund.

TABLE OF CONTENTS

INTRODUCTION	i
STUDY GUIDE	xvii
Account aging	1
Accounts, payable and receivable	2
Alternative minimum tax	3
Amortization/depreciation	4
Annuity	5
Asset protection - limiting liability	6
Bankruptcy	7
Broker, full service and discount	8
Budgets - spending discipline	9
Capital gains	10
Car leasing	11
Cash-flow vs balance sheet	12
Certificate of deposit (CD)	13
Charitable contributions	14
Collection of fees	15
Commercial patents	16
Computers	17
Continuing medical education	18
Cost-of-living adjustment vs merit	19

Creditors - suppliers, IRS	20
Debt - credit, loans	21
Divorce	22
Dollar cost averaging	23
Employee policies and salaries - part-time vs full-time	24
Employee insurance	25
Employment arrangements - solo, partnerships, corporations, institutions	26
Equity - Shareholder's	27
Estate tax	28
Financial advisers - lawyers, accountants, CFP	29
Fringe benefits	30
Gift tax	31
Health proxy (living will)	32
Income - salary vs earnings	33
Incorporation	34
Insurance - disability	35
Insurance - health	36
Insurance - life	37
Interest, simple and compound	38
Interest and dividends	39
Investment-I. stocks and bonds	40

Investment-II. risks and returns	41
Investment-III. growth vs income	42
Investment-IV. rental real estate	43
Investment-V. real estate trusts	44
Investment-VI. types vs age	45
Investment-VII. Treasury securities	46
Investments - "Steinman's Rules"	47
Joint ownership	48
Lawsuits, professional and personal	49
Liquidity	50
Loans, short and long term	51
Long-term medical care	52
Malpractice - definition	53
Malpractice insurance - occurrence vs claims-made	54
Managed care vs indemnity insur.	55
Margin buying	56
Markets, bull and bear	57
Money market funds	58
Mortgage, closing costs	59
Mortgage, fixed and variable rate	60
Municipal bond - tax exemption	61
Mutual funds - open, closed, load, no-load	62

Net worth - personal	63
Office space - rent, sublet, buy	64
Office improvements	65
Options, puts and calls	66
Pension (qualified deferred income)	67
Ratings - bonds and insurance companies	68
Record keeping	69
Roth IRA	70
Savings, insured	71
Savings, types	72
Stock exchange	73
Tax deductible expenses	74
Trusts	75
Uniform Transfers to Minors Act	76
Vesting	77
Vicarious liability	78
Wills - structure	79
Wills - fiduciaries	80
Withholding tax	81
Zero-coupon security	82
POSTSCRIPT	83
INDEX	A

xvii

STUDY GUIDE:

SUBJECTS BY TOPIC

→ See details on pages that follow. ←

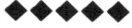

STUDY GUIDE

I. INSURANCE

1) LIFE INSURANCE - P.37
2) DISABILITY INSURANCE - P.35
3) HEALTH INSURANCE - P.36
4) MALPRACTICE INSURANCE P.54
5) MANAGED CARE - P.55
6) RATINGS - P.68

STUDY GUIDE

II. INVESTMENTS

1) BUDGETS - P.9
2) TYPES - PP.40-47
3) MONEY MARKET FUNDS P.58
4) SAVINGS - PP.71-2
5) MUNICIPAL BONDS - P.61
6) MARKETS - P.57
7) MUTUAL FUNDS - P.62
8) CERTIFICATE OF DEPOSIT - P.13
9) ANNUITY - P.5
10) DOLLAR COST AVERAGING - P.23
11) STOCK EXCHANGES - P.73
12) BROKERS - P.8

xx

STUDY GUIDE

III. ASSET PROTECTION

1) LIMITING LIABILITY - p.6
2) CREDITORS - p.20
3) DIVORCE - p.22
4) WILLS - pp.79-80
5) TRUSTS - p.75

STUDY GUIDE

IV. OFFICE MANAGEMENT

1) OFFICE SPACE - pp. 64-5
2) RECORD KEEPING - p. 69
3) COMPUTERS - p. 17
4) COLA VS MERIT - p. 19
5) EMPLOYEE INSURANCE pp. 24-5
6) FRINGE BENEFITS p. 30
7) EMPLOYMENT - p. 26
8) ACCOUNT AGING - p. 1
9) LOANS - p. 51
10) CAR LEASING - p. 11
11) CREDITORS (EQUIPMENT) - p. 20

STUDY GUIDE

V. PERSONAL FINANCE

1) BUDGET - P.9
2) DEBT - P.21
3) FINANCIAL ADVISORS - P.29
4) INCOME - P.33
5) INSURANCE - P.35-7
6) LAWSUITS - P.49
7) BANKRUPTCY - P.7
8) CAPITAL GAINS - P.10
9) NET WORTH - P.63
10) MORTGAGE - PP.59,60

STUDY GUIDE

VI. TAXES

1) ESTATE TAX - P.28
2) GIFT TAX - P.31
3) EXPENSES - P.74
4) WITHHOLDING TAX - P.81

STUDY GUIDE

VII. PENSION

1) QUALIFIED DEFERRED INCOME - p.67
2) VESTING - p.77
3) ANNUITY - p.5
4) ASSET PROTECTION - p.6
5) ROTH IRA - p.70

ACCOUNT AGING

PURPOSE: A bookkeeping method for ascertaining how long a charge has gone unpaid.

METHOD: Each charge for services rendered that has not been paid at the time of service must be charted. Whether done by hand or by computer, it is usual to divide unpaid accounts into groups:
1-30 d   31-60 d   61-90 d   > 90 d
old. At least once a month all outstanding accounts should be aged and rebilling of the patient or his insurance instituted. Once an account surpasses 90 days and rebilling has not been productive, payment is unlikely and collection services (an attorney or a specialized agency) should be considered (see Collection of fees).

ALTERNATIVES: To avoid a systematic collection method will result in significantly lower income and a cash flow problem.

ACCOUNTS PAYABLE/RECEIVABLE

PAYABLE: Amounts owed to creditors and suppliers for goods and services. Typically, a supplier will allow 15 or 30 days for payment once the product is received. Payment within 10 days may gain a 2% discount in some cases. On the other hand, to delay payment may jeopardize future credit and timely delivery following ordering.

RECEIVABLE: Money owed to you for services rendered or goods supplied by you. A delay in receiving payment may require loans to satisfy outstanding bills or payroll on time.

ALTERNATIVE MINIMUM TAX

PURPOSE: Following the Tax Reform Act of 1986, high income individuals, whose predominant itemized deductions against income were from such sources as certain tax shelters and charitable contributions of appreciated property, were no longer able to avoid all taxation.

SIGNIFICANCE: Although most physicians will not commonly be in an income position for the Alternative Minimum Tax (AMT) to be of use, a Federal return must show that regular taxation will result in a higher tax bill than the AMT.

AMORTIZATION/DEPRECIATION

***AMORTIZATION*:** Installments toward retirement of a self-liquidating loan are calculated to pay off the principal and the interest generated in the interim by a selected date (term). In the early years of the repayment, most goes for interest since the principal only decreases by small amounts. In the later years, the bulk of the installment primarily decreases the remaining principal. Thus, with a personal mortgage, for example, the tax deductibility is greatest in the early years of the loan.

***DEPRECIATION*:** The cost value of an asset (e.g., car, equipment) is gradually deducted in segments for tax purposes over its useful life.

ANNUITY

PURPOSE: For the present payment of premiums an insurance company contracts to pay the insured (annuitant) sums of money at a future date (also see Trusts).

ADVANTAGES: Earnings on moneys invested are accumulated tax-deferred. Future income is assured and fixed by the terms of the contract and the financial strength of the insurance company (see Ratings). Annuities are most suitable for people without heirs who seek assured income for the rest of their lives. A special case is a reverse annuity mortgage, where a bank provides lifelong fixed income to an elderly property holder in exchange for gaining title to his house at death.

DISADVANTAGES: Early withdrawals are penalized. Such vehicles are not good protection against future inflation. Reliable individual investments can often yield higher returns (see Investments). Earnings are reduced by insurance company fees.

ASSET PROTECTION - LIMITING LIABILITY EXPOSURE

PURPOSE: to shield assets from creditors and law suits, and to save estate taxes and probate costs.

METHODS: 1) Other than divorce or the IRS, *qualified pension plans* cannot be invaded by creditors (see Pension).

2) *Limited Liability Companies* (LLC) and *Family Limited Partnerships* (FLP), where family members are participants of an entity, shield individual member's other assets from attack of LLC or FLP creditors.

3) *Irrevocable Trusts*, which pass assets to other people (e.g., children), and Foreign Asset Protection Trusts ("offshore trusts") are legal and protect estates, provided they are not created when suits have already been filed or are contemplated.

4) *Transfer* to a spouse or other trusted person.

DISADVANTAGES: Irrevocable transfer of assets to other people permanently removes them from your account (see Divorce, Bankruptcy, Liability, and Trusts).

BANKRUPTCY

PURPOSE: Diminish pressure from creditors to allow discharge or reorganization of debt when obligations overwhelm means.

TYPES (Chapter):

7 - *Liquidation*: all debt is canceled but all non-exempt assets are lost (e.g., in New York State a home is protected only up to $10,000).

11 - *Reorganization:* Court protects assets but oversees debt repayment plan.

DISADVANTAGE: Future credit may be difficult to obtain. Reputation is affected. Legal costs can be significant.

PREVENTION: Disciplined budgeting will keep income in line with life style. When debt becomes large, directly dealing with creditors for rescheduling may alleviate need for legal action.

BROKER, STOCK

PURPOSE: an agent who serves to execute orders to buy or sell equity assets in the market.

TYPES:
Discount: only executes orders and usually furnishes price quotations.

Full service: provides order execution as well as expert advice on offerings and research services to make trading decisions.

ADVANTAGE: For investors who make their own investment decisions, discount trade commissions generate substantial savings, which significantly enhance profits. On the other hand, investors who would benefit from experienced guidance should use full service brokers (see Investment, Mutual Funds).

BUDGETS

PURPOSE: a projected financial plan which balances anticipated income and expenditures for a specified period, based on past history.

ADVANTAGES: Although unexpected adjustments may be needed periodically, general adherence to a budget has revenues cover expenditures. This allows for an orderly flow of cash and a steady rise in net worth. A realistic estimate of earnings and expenses creates a stable economic and social environment.

METHOD: A summation of total income over a specific period of time (e.g., previous year), an estimate of expected income increase in the current period, and a projection of recurrent, periodic, and incidental expenses can be matched and equated. Included in this should be a fixed percentage for savings.

CAPITAL GAINS

DEFINITION: The difference in value between an assets's selling price and its adjusted purchase price.

ADVANTAGES: The maximum long-term capital gains tax rate is presently set at 20%. A distinction is made between assets held more or less than 18 months. With a home (used as a primary residence for 2 of the last 5 years), the calculation is based on the selling price minus the original purchase price and all subsequent value-increasing improvements (with a lifetime exclusion of up to $500,000 for a married couple). The intent of a fixed rate often below an individual's ordinary income tax rate is to encourage capital investments.

CAR LEASING

PURPOSE: Leasing a car sets the fixed monthly costs and guarantees a "buyer" at the end of lease term (either the lessee who has a buyout option or the leasing company which receives the car in return).

DECISION: The portion of expenses, interest, and depreciation related to business use of a car, leased or purchased, is tax deductible. Whether to lease or buy a car is determined by loan finance rate, monthly payments (lease vs buy), charges for excess miles driven, expected trade-in value, anticipated investment earnings on money saved, and "wear-and-tear" charges.

Least expensive: outright purchase without financing.

Next most economical: purchase with financing.

Most expensive: leasing.

CASH-FLOW VS BALANCE SHEET

PURPOSE: To illustrate the distinction between the two concepts shows why, for example, a particular practice may have a large patient load but be caught short of money at critical times.

CASH FLOW: The flow of funds into and out of the practice during a selected accounting period (e.g., first half of January) defined by source and uses of cash.

BALANCE SHEET: Statement of financial position (assets and liabilities) at a particular point in time (e.g., 1/31). Thus, a balance sheet may look like there was enough money available to cover expenses throughout January but in fact there may not yet have been enough funds collected by 1/15 to pay a bill due 1/16.

CERTIFICATE OF DEPOSIT (CD)

PURPOSE: To deposit money with a bank or other financial institution for a specified period of time (weeks to years) to earn interest at a fixed rate.

ADVANTAGES: Since the investment rate of return is set for the life of the CD, the depositor knows his ultimate income at the conclusion, in contrast to other savings accounts whose rates may change daily. The interest rate increases as the term selected increases. Funds are Federally insured. At completion, CD's are renewable.

DISADVANTAGES: CD interest rates are often lower than with other fixed income investments (see Bonds). There are penalties for early withdrawal. Interest is fully taxable.

CHARITABLE CONTRIBUTIONS

PURPOSE: Donations of money or goods to benefit IRS approved organizations engaged in religious, educational, or philanthropic activities.

ADVANTAGES: Donations are usually tax deductible. In particular, a remainder trust allows the donor to receive earnings from his securities as well as a charitable tax deduction while alive; upon death they revert to the charity. This avoids capital gains taxation on securities which may have increased markedly in value with time.

COLLECTION OF FEES

PURPOSE: Fees represent the payment by patients for services rendered (see Accounts Receivable).

METHOD: With cash patients, payment at the time of service is preferred. Delayed billing is more likely to result in some cases of default. With insurance coverage, claims should be submitted as soon after the time of service as possible so that payments can be expected sooner to cover Accounts Payable. An aging schedule (see Account Aging) provides a record of unpaid balances, so that resubmission of claims can be made expeditiously. Medicare in particular insists that deductibles and copayments be pursued actively or the original amount billed would be questioned.

COMMERCIAL PATENTS

REQUIREMENTS:
1) *Novelty* - new and clearly different from the prior art.
2) *Nonobviousness* - inventive idea which is not obvious from just a review of prior art.
3) *Utility* - performs a useful function.

PURPOSE: A Federal Government entitlement to exclude others from employing a newly claimed process, machine, manufacture, or composition of matter ("intellectual property") in the U.S. for 17 years from issue. Foreign protection is also obtainable. Owner of the patent may retain the rights to the invention himself or license its use to another entity. In contradistinction, copyright protection relates to published works and runs for the life of the author plus 50 years.

COMPUTERS

PURPOSE: Computers are central to the operation of an efficient office for billing, patients' records, correspondence, appointment scheduling, account aging, income projections, tax matters, and claims submission.

METHODS: For those not familiar with computer operations, experts can set up and troubleshoot suitable systems. However, learning to do it yourself is much less expensive. Software programs are available to perform all common medical office functions and to network between offices (e.g., Medisoft®). In spite of startup costs, a functional system should be in place from the beginning of operations since data transfer later can be time consuming. Computers routinely come with operating systems which are easy for the novice to negotiate. On line banking programs aid cash flow operations (e.g., Quicken®, Money®).

CONTINUING MEDICAL EDUCATION

PURPOSE: With new discoveries and treatment protocols, it is incumbent upon the practitioner to undertake a regular program of conference attendance and literature review.

METHODS: Teaching hospitals routinely have regular conferences for continuing medical education. Video and audio recordings are available as supplements. Although tax deductible, travel to regional or national meetings can impose a significant cost to the young doctor, with local conferences being comparably productive.

COLA VS MERIT

PURPOSE: Employees expect periodic salary increases which may be determined by cost-of-living adjustments (COLA) or merit, productivity, and profit.

COLA: In the early years of practice, a doctor commonly experiences a delay in developing his patient load until his reputation is established in the community. An employee pay raise keyed to inflation (COLA) may not parallel gross practice income, thus disproportionately increasing overhead expenses.

MERIT: Employees in a new practice should be made to feel that their contributions are key to developing the patient load. Expectations of merit and profit sharing increases at a later date can help to offset this early disadvantage (see Employee Salaries).

CREDITORS

SUPPLIERS: The purchase of equipment for a new office imposes a significant debt load for a new practice. Alternatives can be a financing or rental arrangement with suppliers, with subsequent buy options. Also, use of equipment or furniture from other discontinued practices can meet this initial need.

IRS: The Tax Collector is also amenable to payment plans when the tax payer is unable to make timely installments (see Withholding Tax).

APPROACH: As noted in the Introduction, every physician must avoid excessively expanding debt early in his practice since creditors can sue to invade his private property (see Asset Protection). A balanced program of budgeting outlays against income should be instituted instead.

DEBT

PURPOSE: Money owed another for goods or services rendered, usually formalized by an instrument which stipulates installment amount, interest charges, and due date (term).

ADVANTAGES: Loans or credit are sometimes needed to allow present acquisition of needed supplies to generate future income. If money is required temporarily for operation costs, lenders may require commitment of collateral (owned property of value) to insure repayment. Credit is extended when loan repayment can be expected within a reasonably short period of time.

DISADVANTAGES: Proper budgeting requires that installments must be made on time or additional charges or default may result. If estimates of anticipated income were unrealistic, credit unworthiness may block future applications. Avoid credit card debt since the interest rate is usually very high.

DIVORCE

SIGNIFICANCE: Other than health problems or liability suits, divorce is the greatest risk to a doctor's financial security. Even before an active practice is established, courts can assign value to the anticipated earning potential of a medical degree. Other than non-tax deductible child support, alimony, although tax deductible, may amount to a large part of a doctor's future earnings for many years. Even though most people do not enter a marriage expecting it to end in divorce, in the United States today such is the case 50% of the time.

PROTECTION: Drafted before animosities can affect reasoning, a legally prepared written prenuptial agreement stipulates what property each spouse will receive upon divorce. This will shorten the separation negotiations and keep legal fees down. Irrevocable trusts are another possibility (see Trusts, Asset Protection). Pensions are not shielded. Interspousal property transfer in a divorce is free of tax.

DOLLAR COST AVERAGING

PURPOSE: An investment method whereby a fixed amount of dollars is invested at set intervals (e.g., monthly). Thereby, more shares are bought when the price is low and fewer shares when the price is high. The overall cost would be lower or higher if a fixed number of shares were purchased each time.

ADVANTAGES: Savings are programmed to be made regularly. Assets and net worth accumulate steadily.

DISADVANTAGES: Unless care is taken to regularly monitor the quality of securities being purchased, a market change can reduce the value of the investment portfolio already acquired.

EMPLOYEE INSURANCE

PURPOSE: Under current law, insurance policies must be maintained covering *workmen's compensation* (at work injuries) and *disability* (off work problems).

ADVANTAGES: On-the-job liability is covered and labor laws are satisfied. Employees are aware that their interests are being considered.

DISADVANTAGES: Insurance premiums add to practice overhead. Therefore, the number of employees and the total hours worked should be kept to the minimum needed for efficient operation.

EMPLOYEE POLICIES

METHODS: To avoid misunderstandings, a handbook of employment rules should be given to each new worker, specifying work hours, vacations, sick leave, overtime, coworker relations, duties, standards, benefits, and separation procedures (see COLA vs merit). Employee signs acknowledgment upon receipt of the manual. Computer programs are available for this purpose.

CLASSES: Employees working less than 1000 hours per year are classified as *part-time* and are not necessarily entitled to medical, dental, loan, and pension benefits, whereas *full-time* employees are. Because of this, part-time workers are usually paid more per hour. Especially for working mothers or those holding other jobs, part-time employment may be preferred.

EMPLOYMENT ARRANGEMENTS

SOLE PROPRIETORSHIP: This permits the doctor to make his own policy decisions. He is responsible for all his acts and must arrange coverage when he is unavailable. Initially, income is lower than with groups, but eventually may be more, since overhead is commonly less.

PARTNERSHIP: Cross-coverage is in place but each is responsible for the acts of his partners. (However, see Vicarious Liability; Asset Protection.) Personalities should be compatible. Income distribution must be agreeable to all. Partners are taxed, not the partnership.

CORPORATION: Personal assets are shielded from suits except for malpractice claims. Loans and benefits are available to members. Managerial duties are fulfilled by administrative staff. Group policies, usually established by majority rule, are applicable to all members.

INSTITUTIONS: Employment of doctors by public or private bodies is becoming more common. Salaried physicians satisfy their stipulated work hours and are then free of operational responsibilities beyond that. Generally, income is lower than in private practice.

EQUITY - SHAREHOLDER'S

DEFINITION: Share of ownership in a corporation in the form of stocks bought and possessed by investors, as well as retained earnings (see Investments).

ADVANTAGES: This allows the shareholder of a public corporation voting rights in selecting the Board of Directors and in making charter decisions but does not convey control over the day-to-day operations of the corporation. Equity in public corporations can usually be traded with other investors on the open market without agreement by the company. An investor's personal property is not subject to suits filed against the corporation, except in the case of a professional corporation (see Malpractice).

ESTATE TAX

PURPOSE: The tax imposed by state and federal governments on the assets one owns at the time of death.

DETAILS: Transfers to a surviving spouse are totally tax-free. For other beneficiaries, the first $625,000 (as of 1998) is excluded from taxation. A trust may be established before death whereby estate taxes can be funded by a life insurance policy (see Wills, Trusts). Assets gifted to others (see UTMA and Gift Tax) or transferred irrevocably to a trust during life may be exempt from taxation.

FINANCIAL ADVISERS

PURPOSE: In that laymen are not fully knowledgeable in all aspects of investment and the law, certain advisers should be consulted before making major financial decisions. Selection of candidates can depend on reputation and recommendations from colleagues.

Lawyers: Attorneys may be generalists or experts in specific areas of law (e.g., taxation, malpractice, estate planning, and asset protection).

Accountants: The doctor whose sole income is salary and whose deductions are standard can usually process his own taxes, especially with computer programs now available. More complicated practices, because of periodic changes in the law and the complexity of business returns, need to utilize a certified public accountant (CPA).

Certified Financial Planners: CFP's must pass a qualifying exam demonstrating their ability to advise on financial planning, insurance, banking, investment and taxes. The most objective CFP is usually one who charges a set hourly fee rather than a commission on execution of suggested transactions.

Pension Plan Administrators.

FRINGE BENEFITS

PURPOSE: To compensate full-time employees in addition to salary.

METHODS:

1) Health care - an incorporated practice can cover the costs for treatment and insurance, as long as it does not favor top management preferentially.

2) Personal loans, with fixed term and conditions for repayment (usually at a rate lower than that available from lending institutions).

3) Travel expenses, including job related auto use.

4) Group life insurance.

5) Course to augment professional skills.

6) Pension and profit sharing.

7) Uniform allowance.

GIFT TAX

PURPOSE: A graduated tax imposed on a living donor when the value of the gift exceeds $10,000 per year per donee. Gifts to spouses and charities are exempt and unlimited.

ADVANTAGES: As part of estate planning, money or assets may be passed to children (or anyone else) directly or through a trust while the donor is alive. The total fair market value may be up to $20,000 each and every year (for a donor couple). Interest, dividends, and capital gains of donated assets are taxed at the child's lower rate. Gifts for funding educational or medical expenses incur no tax when made directly to the institution. In this way, estate tax and probate are also avoided at the donor's death (see Wills, UTMA, and Estate Tax).

HEALTH PROXY

PURPOSE: An instrument created before the onset of major illness to define your wishes about any care limitations desired.

ADVANTAGES: A health proxy ("living will") conveys the individual's desires to those directing medical care when a terminal or incapacitating illness or injury occurs, so that indecision in determining an appropriate plan of management can be avoided. Also, the possible postmortem donation of organs should be addressed. In addition, before the need arises, a Power of Attorney should be given to a selected surrogate who is not a beneficiary of your will (e.g., a relative, friend, attorney, or bank) to manage your financial affairs responsibly if and when you are disabled.

DISADVANTAGES: Stipulations may not conform with good medical practice in certain prescribed situations.

INCOME

SALARY: This is the amount of money paid to you by your practice for services rendered. To aid budgeting, the monthly amount should be the same during a given year. Tax rates (brackets) are graduated and vary with total amount earned in the year.

EARNINGS: This is the amount remaining from practice income after paying expenses and staff salaries. The net may be retained for future use, applied to the purchase of equipment or satisfaction of a loan, given as bonuses, or distributed to a pension plan if profit sharing is elected. Retained earnings are taxed to the practice in the year received. If distributed to shareholders of a corporation as dividends, they are taxed to them as ordinary income.

INCORPORATION

PURPOSE: to shield shareholder's personal assets from law suits resulting from the actions of the corporation and its employees as well as product liability.

ADVANTAGES: Establishment of an uncomplicated corporation can be executed with do-it-yourself kits (e.g., Blumberg Pub., NYC) and helpful state offices, thus saving legal fees. To maintain the corporation as a distinct legal entity, certain formalities such as separate checking, a formal charter, stationery, and minutes of annual meetings are needed. Employees have special benefit options (see Fringe Benefits). A "Subchapter S" entity combines the protection of a corporation and the tax benefits of a partnership.

DISADVANTAGES: Professional corporations (PC) do not shield personal assets from malpractice suits, no longer give extra pension advantages, and require all shareholders to be licensed in the profession.

INSURANCE - DISABILITY

PURPOSE: Prolonged disability of the key wage-earner without alternative income poses a bigger threat to family financial security than death, since cash input stops <u>and</u> the disabled also requires ongoing maintenance. Continuing income assurance is essential from the startup of practice.

METHOD: Insurance coverage is available for various waiting periods of disability (e.g., 28, 60, 90 days). Applications should detail the most technically demanding aspects of one's professional activities (<u>not</u> generalized). Coverage should be continued until sizeable savings are attained. Amount of coverage should be enough to maintain a family in a reasonable style, not just subsistence. For health-related disability starting after age 50, most policies only cover until age 65. Benefits are taxable if premiums were paid by the employer.

INSURANCE - HEALTH

PURPOSE: to cover the costs of medical care, especially prolonged illnesses.

METHOD: Professional courtesy can no longer be counted on to cover medical costs. Also, emergency care and hospitalization are expensive and must be paid. In addition to a basic policy, catastrophic coverage is essential and is relatively inexpensive. Some employers provide basic health insurance. Tax deductibility of medical costs only begins after large expenditures. Even young doctors sometimes get sick (see Insurance - disability). Along with life and disability, health insurance represents an essential undertaking from the very beginning of practice.

INSURANCE - LIFE

PURPOSE: To provide an instant estate if premature death takes the key wage earner of a family, especially early in his career when savings are small.

TYPES: *Whole life* (including "universal" and "variable" life) - combines a compulsory savings plan with life coverage, thereby generating cash value and a potential loan source. This strategy is good for spendthrifts and for apprehensive investors.
Term life - provides only death benefit with no cash value at conclusion. Savings on lower premium can be invested independently, with potentially higher returns.

ADVANTAGES: To maximize immediate death benefit coverage only, term life is much less expensive. Guaranteed renewability (without exam) and convertibility (to whole life) options are essential. Premiums rise with age. Preexisting conditions are usually not covered, so initiation at a young age is recommended.

INTEREST - TYPES

SIMPLE: The amount paid by a borrower for the use of money for a particular period (e.g., one year). The amount paid in ensuing periods is calculated on the amount of the original principal only.

COMPOUND: Same as simple interest except that the amount paid in the second period is calculated based on the total of the principal and interest accumulated in the first period.

EXAMPLE: If $100 is borrowed at 12% annual interest, payable once a year, both simple and compound interest yield a total of $112 at the end of the first year. After two years, assuming no decrease in principal, simple interest produces a total of $124 whereas compounding totals $125.44. By the "Rule of 72" (72/12=6), $100 will double to $200 in six years by compounding, whereas simple interest accumulation yields $172.

INTEREST/DIVIDENDS

INTEREST: The amount paid by a borrower for the use (rental) of money for a specific time period (see Interest). The amount is fixed by the stipulations of the loan.

DIVIDENDS: Distribution of company earnings to shareholders. Except for preferred stock, the amount paid is variable and is set by profitability and alternative uses of profits (see Investments - stocks and bonds).

ATTRIBUTES: Both dividends and interest are taxable as ordinary income.

INVESTMENTS -
I. STOCKS AND BONDS

STOCKS:
Preferred - No voting rights. Dividends are at a rate fixed at time of original issue. Payment of dividends takes priority over common stock. Share prices change more gradually than common stock. There is never repayment of principal. Shares are traded on the open market. Yield is typically higher than with bonds. Usually offered by utilities.

Common - Typically coveys voting rights. If the company is very profitable, dividends may be larger than with preferred stock. Share prices are more volatile and, over time, normally attain greater appreciation than other forms of investment.

BONDS:
Evidence of an issuer's indebtedness on which the bondholder receives interest for the use of his money. Bonds can be traded like stocks and fluctuate in price. Bonds may be redeemed ("called") by the issuer on specific dates before maturity if interest rates fall.

INVESTMENTS -
II. RISKS AND RETURNS

PURPOSE: A well-conceived investment plan balances risk against reward (see Capital gains, Interest/dividends).

METHOD: There is always a tradeoff between risks and returns - the higher the risk, the higher the possible return on investment, and vice versa. Personal savings and pensions should be confined to relatively safe securities. Bonds are rated by Moody's and by Standard and Poor's services for credit risk (AAA and AA are of highest quality and safety). Federal and federally insured securities have the lowest risk.

INVESTMENT -
III. GROWTH VS INCOME

PURPOSE: Stocks can be classified by their potential for long-term above-average asset growth (appreciation) versus current income from dividends. Certain types of investments are classically known for *growth* (e.g., stock of large established companies with low dividends) versus *income* (e.g., high-dividend preferred securities of utilities).

METHOD: The selection of investments in a portfolio should balance the need for current supplies of money, safety, and planning for future requirements (see Mutual Funds, Stocks and bonds, Savings).

INVESTMENT -
IV. RENTAL REAL ESTATE

PURPOSE: Although one's own home is in most cases the largest single investment made by individuals, purchase of rental property can augment other sources of income.

ADVANTAGES: Desirable property (homes or apartments) can be selected for current income potential and long-term capital appreciation (see Capital gains). Asset depreciation and maintenance have business tax advantages.

DISADVANTAGES: Income is lost but overhead outlays continue during periods of vacancy. Investment in repairs and periodic refurbishing is required to maintain value. Liability for tenant actions must be covered and exposes landlord to attack (see Asset Protection). Timely collection of rents and eviction of nonpaying or uncooperative tenants is sometimes a problem.

INVESTMENT -
V. REAL ESTATE TRUSTS

PURPOSE: An investment portfolio which includes various real estate purchases yielding rental receipts, mortgage income, and capital gains from sales (REIT).

ADVANTAGES: As with any collective trust, REIT's utilize large money pools from several investors to deal with major projects and diversified offerings. This dilutes risk, decreases costs, and expands investment opportunities which an individual investor might not otherwise be able to consider. Professional management increases the chance of profitable and timely investments. The individual is shielded from legal misfortunes of the trust. On the other hand, earnings of the trust pass through to each investor.

INVESTMENT -
VI. TYPES VS AGE

PURPOSE: A young practitioner may consider investments with somewhat more inherent risk since he has more years to cover judgment errors. As the investor approaches retirement, less risk can be allowed.

METHOD: Stocks may be a large part of the portfolio of the younger investor. Safe fixed income and liquid securities (bonds, CD's, annuities, money market funds, and Federal Government obligations) should dominate holdings in later years. All individuals, regardless of age, may want to keep an amount in cash, precious metals, or liquid assets to cover unexpected short term needs (see Liquidity, Savings, Treasury Securities). Fixed income securities (e.g., bonds) generally yield smaller long-term returns than stocks.

INVESTMENT -
VII. TREASURY SECURITIES

PURPOSE: Savings in U.S. Government paper represent the safest of all investments. Purchased through brokers or directly from any Federal Reserve office. Other than savings bonds, they are sold at competitive auction. Non-competing purchases are sold at the average price of winning bids. The longer the term of the investment, the higher is the rate of interest. At maturity, funds may be reinvested in new offerings. All are exempt from state and local tax.

TYPES: *Bills* - short-term securities with maturities of one year or less, most commonly 91 or 182 days.
 Notes - maturities of 1-10 years.
 Bonds - maturities of >10 years.
 Savings bonds - low denomination bonds sold in banks at discount and redeemed before term or at maturity at prevailing rates, but for no more than 6% interest. Appreciated Series E bonds can be exchanged for HH bonds tax free, thus deferring taxation of accumulated interest.

INVESTMENTS - "STEINMAN'S GUIDELINES"

1) Never accept advice blindly - research your own investment decisions before execution.
2) Never give advice.
3) Never fall in love with a failing security (divorce is better than suicide).
4) Your money should be working maximally for you at all times through diversification.
5) Check the performance of your holdings at least twice a week.
6) Determining when to sell a stock is the toughest of all decisions.
7) Never look back.
8) Money in hand is worth more than on paper.
9) Learn and refine how to manage your finances as diligently as you learned how to manage your patients.
10) Investing is a tool for achieving long-term economic security for your family, as much as your practice income is.

Suggested references:
1) Value Line Investment Survey
2) Forbes Stock Market Course

JOINT OWNERSHIP

PURPOSE: A means for two or more people to hold property or assets together which avoids probate on death, making needed assets available without legal costs or delays.

TYPES: 1) *Tenancy in common* - When one owner dies, his undivided interest passes to a designated heir.

2) *Joint tenancy with right of survivorship* - One owner may sell his interest without approval of the other(s). When one owner dies, his interest passes to the other owner(s).

3) *Tenancy by the entirety* - For married couples only. Ownership cannot be transferred without the other's consent. When one dies, his/her interest passes to the other spouse. Converts to a tenancy in common upon divorce.

LAWSUITS - PROFESSIONAL AND PERSONAL

PROFESSIONAL: Actions while performing medical functions must be covered by appropriate insurance; generally $1m/$3m is minimal protection today. Personal holdings must be shielded separately (see Asset Protection). Actions which are illegal or unethical are not covered (also see Vicarious Liability, Malpractice). A separate policy for non-profession-related events within your office (e.g., falls) must be arranged.

PERSONAL: Liability potential for all members of your household must be covered. This includes events relating to use of home and car. An "umbrella" policy for $1m - $3m (above basic coverage) should be purchased to protect against large claims and is relatively inexpensive but essential.

LIQUIDITY

DEFINITION: Resources or assets which are easily convertible to cash, such as money market funds, U.S. Treasury bills, an existing credit line, and bank deposits (see Savings).

PURPOSE: Such funds should be immediately accessible in case of unanticipated emergency, illness, disability, appearance of a desirable investment, or timely satisfaction of debt. Cash should be enough to cover at least one month of expenses. This level of assurance will maintain good credit ratings and permit taking advantage of new market opportunities, which is especially important if there is a temporary slowdown in cash inflow. Budgets should not be so closely defined as to overlook the possibility of departures from expected receipts.

LOANS

PURPOSE: The allowance by a lender for a borrower to use property or money for a specified period of time, after which the asset is returned with interest paid for its use.

SHORT-TERM: For the temporary use of an asset, credit can be established guaranteeing the return or repayment of the loan. Credit card loans, although easily obtained, commonly have the highest rate of interest, making it desirable to pay current balances when due rather than incurring interest charges for delayed remittance.

LONG-TERM: These loans usually require execution of a written agreement in which the conditions are specified. Other than mortgage and home equity loans, personal debt interest is not tax-deductible.

LONG-TERM MEDICAL CARE

PURPOSE: Preplanning is necessary to anticipate large outlays related to prolonged and/or terminal illness and disability.

COVERAGE: A policy covering catastrophic illnesses is essential to prevent exhausting savings. In addition, new legislation prohibits the rapid transfer of assets in anticipation of Medicaid coverage for terminal nursing home care. The gradual irrevocable transfer of assets (see Asset Protection, Trusts) with the grantor as income beneficiary well before the onset of illness helps in qualifying for Medicaid insurance should the need arise.

MALPRACTICE - DEFINITION

CUSTOMARY: Negligence in the exercise of a professional function, whether intended or not, which departs from expected diligence and ordinary skill according to accepted medical practices. (Incomplete record keeping may give the incorrect impression of negligent care or attitude.)

CRITERIA: 1) A relationship exists between doctor and patient whereby a *duty* to perform a service is established;

2) A *breach* in the performance of that duty occurs, as measured by applicable standards of care;

3) Monetary or physical *damages* to the patient result from the breach; and

4) A proximate cause-and-effect relationship (*causation*) between the performance and the damage can be identified.

MALPRACTICE INSURANCE

PURPOSE: to provide coverage in the event of lawsuits related to professional functions. Premiums are tax-deductible business expenses.

OCCURRENCE: This policy is in effect for the duration of the Statute of Limitations for delayed initiation of a suit. Premiums are higher than claims-made. Indemnity remains in effect for events taking place during the coverage period even after termination of the policy. In the absence of tort reform, it is likely that premiums will continue to rise in the foreseeable future.

CLAIMS-MADE: Events are covered only if the suit is filed in the incident year when the policy is active. Additional "tail" coverage is needed for suits filed later. Initially, premiums for the basic policy are lower than the occurrence type but eventually rise in the subsequent years the policy is continued.

MANAGED CARE VS INDEMNITY INSURANCE

COMPARISON: Traditionally, indemnity (commercial) health insurance covered nearly all claims for benefits submitted by any physician the patient may choose. Managed care (e.g., HMO) requires referral of patients to a specialist by primary care physicians ("gatekeepers") as well as review and precertification by the insurance company for special procedures. With HMO's only the roster of approved physicians may be used, except in emergencies. Roster physicians agree to accept the HMO's contracted reimbursement, which is generally lower than that of indemnity companies. Primary care physicians are paid by capitation, i.e., a fixed biweekly payment regardless of frequency or extent of care, whereas specialists are usually paid on a fee-for-service basis. Some HMO's run their own clinics, with physicians being paid a fixed salary regardless of patient load.

EFFECT: The pool of HMO insureds provides an instant source of new patients. Income projections are clear from the published reimbursements schedules. However, patient care is dictated in part by procedures the HMO is willing to endorse.

MARGIN BUYING

PURPOSE: A means for purchasing securities on credit without putting up the full price (leverage). Interest is charged for this privilege.

ADVANTAGES: The investor must deposit with the broker money or securities to serve as collateral for the loan. If the stock rises, large profits can be made on commitment of small amounts of cash.

DISADVANTAGES: If the stock drops in price, the brokerage may "call" the loan and insist that it be repaid with cash, bank loans, or liquidation of the collateralizing securities, which may themselves be quality investments. Thus, the potential exists for losses larger than the initial purchase amount. Because of the inherent risk, margin buying should not be routinely employed.

MARKETS - BULL/BEAR

DEFINITION: A rising market = *bull*.
A falling market = *bear*.

STRATEGY: As defined by various indices (e.g., Dow Jones Industrial Average - a weighted average of the share price of 30 actively traded large companies), the investor can get a summary picture of market trends. A change in an index may reflect changes in the overall economy. However, if a particular stock is dropping regularly while the index rises, caution against purchase or continued holding of the asset should be exercised. A stock which rises faster than the index should be considered favorable, all other factors being equal. This is scrutinized by regularly charting daily share prices. A one-day change may not forecast a general trend.

MONEY MARKET FUNDS

PURPOSE: An open-ended mutual fund which invests in short-term, highly liquid, safe securities.

ADVANTAGES: The fund's net asset value is kept at $1/share and only the interest rate (and, therefore, the number of shares) changes, based on market conditions. Shares may be redeemed at any time via cash or check writing privileges. Thus, money is readily available when needed. Yields are usually more than a bank savings account. Yield of a particular fund can be measured against the weekly Donoghue Average of all major money market funds.

DISADVANTAGES: After subtracting the fund's management fees, returns on investment are relatively low. Funds are not federally insured. Interest is taxable except for funds based on municipal bonds.

MORTGAGE - CLOSING COSTS

PURPOSE: The acquisition of a mortgage on personal or business property may require the payment of certain expenses at closing.

TYPES: 1) *Legal fees* - the borrower pays for his own and the lender's lawyer.
2) *Appraisal* - to determine if the property is worth the amount requested.
3) *Environmental* - to evaluate absence of asbestos and termites as well as local environmental conditions.
4) *Tax escrow* - reserve to pay future property taxes.
5) *Insurance* - to cover replacement in event of casualty, fire, or flood.
6) *Title insurance* - to be sure that no one has prior claim on the property.
7) *Certificate of occupancy* - certification by municipality that property is fit to use for intended purpose.
9) *Points* - up-front percentage of loan amount added on to cost of the loan.
10) *Application fee* - processing charge (assuming no agent commissions).
11) *Per diem loan interest* paid at closing for the balance of month in which closing occurs.
12) *Mortgage taxes* - state and local fees for establishment of mortgage.

MORTGAGE - FIXED/VARIABLE

PURPOSE: The interest rate may be set at closing or left to vary according to market conditions.

FIXED: By setting the rate at closing it is possible to budget monthly installments for the life of the loan.

VARIABLE: If interest rates are expected to drop, a variable mortgage will result in lower monthly charges; the opposite is also true.

ADVANTAGES: The purchase of a property generates accumulated equity value as the mortgage is paid off. Interest on a home or office loan is tax deductible. Rent for office space, although deductible as a business expense, leaves no asset value at the end of the occupancy period. Rent may be lower than monthly mortgage premiums and property taxes, thus easing cash flow in the early years of a practice. Property equity can be used as collateral in later loan transactions for real estate or personal purchases ("home equity loan"), whose interest is also tax deductible.

MUNICIPAL BONDS - TAX EXEMPT MUNIS

PURPOSE: A fixed-term debt obligation of a state or city government, which is free of federal and, in the state or city of issue, any local income taxes.

ADVANTAGES: Although different "munis" vary in credit strength, they are generally considered safe investments (see Ratings; Investment - Stock and Bonds). Munis are traded through securities brokers and may be sold before maturity on the open market. With investors in high tax brackets, munis yield interest equivalent to other taxable securities with much higher taxable returns. They should not be in the portfolio of a pension (deferred taxation) plan.

DISADVANTAGES: Uninsured munis may default. Like other fixed income investments, a rise in interest rates will decrease the muni's market value.

MUTUAL FUNDS

PURPOSE: A pool of money from individual shareholders managed by an investment company for investing conservatively or aggressively in a large portfolio of stocks, bonds, money market, and other securities. Such funds offer diversification (hence, dilution of risk) and professional management. Fund shares are marketable or redeemable, and returns on investment are taxable to the shareholder.

TYPES: 1) *Open-ended* - new shares are created by the fund in response to market demand from new or current investors.

2) *Closed-ended* - number of shares is limited from the outset.

3) *Load* - sold with an up-front sales charge so that salesman will offer investment advice and an explanation of fund particulars.

4) *No-load* - sold by the fund directly to investors with no up-front sales charge.

NET WORTH - PERSONAL

CALCULATION: Total value of all possessions (accounts receivable, property, investments, pension plan vesting, cash, savings, practice goodwill) minus debts (mortgage, loans, accounts payable).

PURPOSE: Up-to-date knowledge of net worth aids estate planning, application for new loans or investments, budgeting, and cash flow. Net worth at the end of a period minus the beginning should equal net income (or loss) during that time. Equivalent to a shareholder's equity in a corporation. Periodic calculation of net worth will ascertain the increase of an individual's savings for future use.

OFFICE SPACE - RENT, SUBLET, OR BUY

PURPOSE: A suitable work environment is just as important to a successful practice as effective instrumentation.

ADVANTAGES: 1) *Rent* - For the new doctor, startup funds are usually adequate only to lease office space, thereby keeping monthly property expenses manageable. Conditions are limited by landlord rules and preexisting layout. Rent is deducted as a current expense. Property has no asset value to the tenant at the end of the lease.

2) *Sublet* - Part-time use of space also employed by another doctor at alternate times economizes on outlays for space and equipment but limits schedule flexibility and individual preferences.

3) *Buy* - If mortgaging will not overextend credit and anticipated receipts are adequate, office purchase allows exercise of individual preferences, expanding equity as mortgage is paid off, depreciation for tax purposes, and patient identification of the unique location of a particular doctor. Property usually appreciates in value with time.

OFFICE IMPROVEMENTS

PURPOSE: Individual design of layout allows maximum usage of space with incorporation of the doctor's tastes and preferences.

ADVANTAGES: Appropriate design of decors, furniture, communications, and patient flow creates efficient operation for when the practice is running on a daily basis. Improvements are tax deductible if they increase potential for income generation. Modifications should always be delineated with the contractor by a formal, written legal agreement. Repair of equipment is also deductible if it adds to the life and value of the property, but not if it only maintains or replaces it with an equivalent. For the new doctor, purchase of used apparatus and furniture from discontinued practices defers major outlays until adequate funds are available for more up-to-date acquisitions. Rental from a supplier or procuring on an installment plan is another possibility.

OPTIONS - PUTS AND CALLS

PURPOSE: Through the purchase of puts or calls ("derivatives"), investments can be executed with lower cash commitments (the cost of the option instead of the cost of the underlying shares).

PUTS: These investment contracts give the holder the right to sell a particular stock to the writer of the option at a fixed price before a specified expiration date. This insures that the share price at the time of sale will not be below the target amount and thus offers downside protection in a bear market.

CALLS: This is an option to buy at a defined price where the seller agrees to deliver a particular stock on a timely basis at the specified figure. If the share cost of the stock is above the strike price, the option buyer profits by the difference. In general, options tend to be speculative and should be avoided by cautious investors. Similarly, most doctors should abstain from short (borrowed) sales.

PENSIONS - QUALIFIED DEFERRED INCOME

PURPOSE: To set aside funds during periods of active employment for later use upon retirement. Current qualified contributions are usually deductible from gross income. Investment income and capital gains taxes are deferred until withdrawal. Early withdrawals may be penalized at 10%. The doctor may manage his own funds or give the responsibility to a financial adviser or broker.

TYPES: 1) *Deferred earned salary* or bonuses - taxed when actually received.

2) *401*(k) - corporate employee pre-tax contributions of salary to a qualified plan, allowing distribution after age 59½.

3) *IRA* - individual retirement savings for employees not otherwise covered by a qualified plan (see Roth IRA).

4) *Keogh* - pension plan for the self-employed.

5) *Defined benefits* - contributions are based on actuarial calculation of amount needed to achieve a target retirement benefit.

6) *Profit sharing* - pension contribution determined by corporate net earnings.

7) *Defined contribution* - contribution fixed as percentage of employee's salary.

8) *Annuities*.

9) *Social Security* (see Withholding).

RATINGS - BONDS AND INSURANCE COMPANIES

PURPOSE: to define for the purchaser the relative risk of employing certain instruments for estate and financial planning.

BONDS: To minimize risk of default, bonds should only be purchased with ratings of AA or AAA by Moody's or Standard and Poor's (see Investment - Risks and Returns).

INSURANCE: Companies are ranked by Best's Rating Service. Top rating is A+. Buyers should consider ratings to ascertain that a company is financially sound, thus assuring coverage if need for payout is ever required (see Insurance). Also, a company's financial rating by Dun and Bradstreet should be evaluated.

RECORD KEEPING

BUSINESS: A standardized register of business transactions aids in monthly bank account reconciliation, budget projections for coming periods, and preparation of tax returns. Single entry bookkeeping, by hand or computer, itemizes income and expense activity (see Computers). If a receptionist collects patient fees, a system must be set up to verify that all receipts are recorded and deposited.

MEDICAL: A legible process for recording patient data and examination findings on each visit is essential (see Malpractice). Written documentation, which should be stored safely for at least seven years, may be needed later to substantiate claims of thorough care.

ROTH IRA

PURPOSE: Created in 1997, this retirement account option allows individuals to accumulate earnings and to ultimately receive distributions income tax-free (see Pension).

CONDITIONS: 1) Can be utilized by those who also participate in another type of qualified retirement plan (e.g., 401(k)).

2) Funded with after-tax dollars.

3) Eligible for up to a $2000 annual contribution, based on adjusted gross income and marital status.

4) May be distributed tax-free after age 59½, at death, or with disability if account has existed for at least 5 years.

5) Lifetime penalty-free limit of $10,000 withdrawal for first-time home purchases.

SAVINGS - INSURED

PURPOSE: In addition to reducing risk by selecting assets by rating systems (see Ratings), it is desirable to invest moneys in insured accounts and securities. The cost for the insurance is usually passed on to the investor in the form of reduced returns.

METHOD: 1) Bank accounts: FDIC (Federal Deposit Insurance Corp.) or FSLIC (Federal Savings and Loan Insurance Corp.)

2) Brokerage accounts: SIPC (Securities Investor Protection Corp.)

3) Municipal bonds: MBIA (Municipal Bond Insurance Assoc.)

4) Credit union accounts: NCUA (National Credit Union Administration)

SAVINGS - TYPES

PURPOSE: To maintain a portion of investments in liquid accounts in case of emergency need.

TYPES: 1) Deposit accounts - deposits in federally insured bank or credit union accounts.
    2) Certificates of Deposit (CD)
    3) U.S. Savings Bonds
    4) Money market funds with check writing privileges.
    5) Cash and precious metals.
    6) Tax-exempt bond fund with check writing privileges, for high income individuals.

CAUTION: To guard family needs before and after death, divide liquid assets between:
    1) a bank safe deposit box (Courts will seal it after death until probate and IRS investigations are completed); and
    2) a joint spousal or "payable-upon-death" account, where assets go to a designated beneficiary without probate of a will (see Joint Ownership, Liquidity).

STOCK EXCHANGE

PURPOSE: An organized marketplace in which stocks and bonds are traded for and by investors. Trading is regulated by the Securities and Exchange Commission (SEC).

TYPES: 1) New York Stock Exchange (*NYSE*): The shares of more than 3000 large companies are traded. This accounts for about 60% of all shares traded on national exchanges.

2) American Stock Exchange (*AMEX*): The shares of small to medium-size companies are traded.

3) Over the Counter (*OTC*): Small company securities not listed on an organized exchange are traded by phone and computer between dealers' offices and monitored by the National Association of Securities Dealers (NASD).

4) Commodities exchanges - Various exchanges organized to trade commodity futures and options.

TAX-DEDUCTIBLE EXPENSES

PURPOSE: Specific personal and business expenses may be itemized for Federal tax deductions, subject to certain limitations. (An accountant or tax attorney should be consulted for a complete listing and applicability to particular situations and tax brackets.)

TYPES:
1) Medical expenses
2) State and local taxes
3) Mortgage interest
4) Charity
5) Casualty and theft losses
6) Expenditures made in generating business activity or perfecting trade skills.

TRUSTS

PURPOSE: A legal relationship where one person (trustee) holds title to property of a donor (grantor) for the benefit of another (beneficiary).

TYPES:

1) *Testamentary trust* - created by a will.

2) *Inter vivos trust* - created while the donor is alive. The donor may enjoy the proceeds of the trust until death (e.g., charitable remainder trust) or may irrevocably gift the trust assets to the beneficiary (see Annuity; Asset Protection; UTMA).

3) *Irrevocable life insurance trust* - pays insured's estate taxes and is protected from creditors (also see Long-term Medical Care).

UNIFORM TRANSFERS TO MINORS

PURPOSE: To provide a means for gifting to minor children (UTMA) whereby a custodian manages the assets until majority or until needed for specific uses (e.g., education, illness).

ADVANTAGES: Interest earned is taxed at the minor's lower tax rate. Investment of the funds is controlled by a responsible adult. Asset is shielded if the donor is sued.

DISADVANTAGE: Under the Tax Reform Act of 1986, annual unearned income (e.g., interest and dividends) in excess of $1200 for children under 14 years of age is taxed at the donor's rate. In a divorce, the tax is calculated at the custodial parent's rate (see Gift tax).

VESTING

PURPOSE: The right of an employee to a percentage of employer-contributed moneys set aside in a qualified pension increases with the years of service and is paid out when he retires or leaves the company (see Pension).

METHODS: Under the Tax Reform Act of 1986, employees must be fully vested after five years of service. A typical vesting schedule would be:

< 2 y - 0%   2 y - 20%   3 y - 40%
 4 y - 60%   5 y - 80%   6 y -100%

Vesting becomes 100% if he reaches retirement age, dies, or is disabled. Upon termination of employment, vested amounts may be distributed as a rollover to another qualified plan (e.g., IRA), to a surviving spouse, or to a retired employee as cash.

VICARIOUS LIABILITY

PURPOSE: When one practitioner relies on another to cover or participate in the care of his patients, the former is responsible in part for the other's actions.

METHOD: Especially in group practices, an insurance rider must be carried by the primary doctor which covers any malpractice caused by a physician's employees (e.g., nurses, physician assistants) or a covering doctor, even though the primary doctor is not on duty or directly treated the patient at the time of the negligent event.

WILLS - STRUCTURE

PURPOSE: A legal document which specifies the distribution of estate probate assets according to the wishes of the deceased.

ADVANTAGES: Everyone should have a will prepared by an experienced lawyer before health problems or creditors appear. If a person dies without a will ("intestate"), assets are distributed according to statutory provision. A will notwithstanding, most states dictate the minimum percentage a surviving spouse receives. If conditions change before death, a new will can be executed, overriding the earlier version.

DISADVANTAGES: A court must pass on the legality of a will before it can be effected, sometimes involving large legal fees and delays of several months. In the interim, beneficiaries may be without resources for daily living (for alternatives, see Trusts, Joint Ownership, Savings, Asset Protection). "Do-it-yourself" kits should be avoided so that complicated issues can be confronted legally.

WILLS - FIDUCIARIES

PURPOSE: A will must specify the persons or institutions (e.g., a bank) who will carry out the wishes of the maker of the will. Otherwise, a probate or surrogate judge will appoint such functionaires.

TESTATOR: The person who executes his will.

BENEFICIARY: Person (heir) receiving real and personal property distributed by the will.

TRUSTEE: The person specified in the will to receive, manage, and distribute assets over a period of time for the benefit of one or more beneficiaries.

EXECUTOR: The person appointed to be sure that the wishes expressed in a will are carried out. This may be the same person as the Trustee. The Court will appoint an Administrator if no Executor is defined by a will or agrees to serve.

GUARDIAN: The person appointed by the deceased to care for his minor children if there is no surviving parent.

WITHHOLDING TAX

PURPOSE: Begun during the Civil War, certain taxes must be deducted regularly from an employee's gross salary and transferred promptly to the government (federal, state, and local) by the employer.

TYPES: 1) *Income tax* - As fixed by the employee's tax bracket, an amount is deducted from gross salary in anticipation of the employee's final year-end total tax liability.

2) *FICA* - Social security retirement fund contribution as a percent of gross salary (currently 6.2%), subject to an annual maximum.

3) *Medicare* - Like FICA, a fixed percentage (currently 1.45%) is withheld, with no annual maximum.

4) *Unemployment tax* - Up to a mandated maximum, the employer usually pays a percentage of his employee's gross salary. Nothing is paid by the employee.

ZERO-COUPON SECURITY

PURPOSE: An investment instrument that is sold at discount, makes no periodic interest payments, appreciates at a preset rate, and is redeemed at face value at term.

ADVANTAGES: Since the IRS taxes interest as accrued each year even though not received, this type of security is recommended for tax-deferred retirement accounts. "Zeros" are commonly used to anticipate specific investment goals such as college tuition or retirement. The longer the term of the security, the lower is the initial discounted purchase price, thus leveraging the investment. Most zeros can be sold on the open market before term.

DISADVANTAGE: Since interim interest is not paid, zeros are usually subject to greater shifts in market value than normal bonds when interest rates rise or fall.

POSTSCRIPT

This text has endeavored to present an introduction into issues that should concern both the new and the established practitioner. It has served its objective if the reader is now broadly aware of the subjects which deserve closer scrutiny and mastery to insure a life of comfort, security, and physical contentment, as a complement and aid to professional achievement.

In summary, the individual must be informed so that he is ultimately the master of his own fate.

"LIFE IS SHORT, THE ART [KNOWLEDGE] LONG, OPPORTUNITY FLEETING, EXPERIENCE TREACHEROUS, JUDGMENT DIFFICULT."

HIPPOCRATES

ANNOUNCEMENT

For educational institutions or special groups that may be interested, the author, Dr. Gary Steinman, is available for lectures on subjects covered by this book. The publisher, Baffin Books, Inc., should be contacted by fax for reservations and details at (718) 278-0354.

◆◆◆◆◆

A

INDEX

Accountant	29,74
Accounts receivable	2,15
Accounts payable	2
Aging, account	1,5
Alimony	22
AMEX	73
Amortization	4
AMT	3
Annuity	5,45,67
Asset protection	6,22,34,49,52,79
Assets	4,8
Balance sheet	12
Bankruptcy	7
Bear market	57
Beneficiary	80
Benefits	25-6,30,34
Billing	1
Bills, investment	46
Bonds	40,45-6,62,68,72
Bonus	33
Bookkeeping	1,12,15,17,29,69
Budget	7,9,21,60,63,69
Bull market	57

B

Calls, investment	66
Capital gains	10,14,31,41,43-4,67
Car leasing	11
Cash flow	9,12
Certificate of Deposit	9,12-3,45,60,72
Certificate of Occupancy	59
Charity	14
Child support	22
Collateral	21,60
Collection of fees	1,15
College education	3,31,70
Commodities	73
Computers	17
Corporation	26,29,34
Credit	7,51,56
Credit cards	21,51
Creditors	6,7,20,48,79
Custodian	76
Debt	7,20-1
Deferred income	67,70
Depreciation	4,43,64
Disability	24,32
Disability insurance	35
Dividend	31,33,39-42
Divorce	6,22,48,76

C

Dollar Cost Averaging	23
Dow Jones Average	57
Earnings	33
Employees	24-5
Employment	26
Equipment	65
Equity	27,60,64
Estate	6,37
Estate planning	16,29,31
Estate tax	6,28
Executor	80
FDIC	71
FICA	81
Financial adviser	29
FSLIC	71
Full-time employees	25
Gifts	28,31,35
Group practice	26
Growth securities	42
Guardian	80
Health proxy ("living will")	32
Health insurance	30,36,52,55
Heirs	5,80
HMO	55
Home	10,43,60,70

D

Home equity loan	51
Income	42-3
Indemnity, insurance	54-5
Institutional employment	26
Insurance	5,15,24,29,30,35,59,68,78
Interest	13,31,38-9,46,58,60,82
Investment	8,13,16,23,27,29,40-7,50,56, 63,66-8,71,73,75,77,82
IRA	67,77
IRS	16,20
Keogh	67
Lawyer	29,59,74
Leverage	16,56
Liability	6,24,30,43,48-9,53,78
Life insurance	30,37,75
Liquidity	45,50,58,72
Loan	2,4,11,21,25,30,33,40,51
Malpractice	34,53,69
Malpractice insurance	54
Managed Care	55
Margin	16,56
MBIA	71
Medical education	18
Medicare, Medicaid	15,52,80
Merit, salary	19

E

Money market	45,58,62,72
Moody's	68
Mortgage	5, 51,59,60,74
Municipal bonds	61
Mutual funds	58,62
NCUA	71
Negligence	53,78
Net worth	63
Notes, investment	46
NYSE	73
Office	17,26,60,64-5
Options, investment	66
Organ donation	32
OTC	73
Ownership	48
Partnerships	26
Part-time employees	25
Patents and copyrights	16
PC	34
Pension	6,22,30,33-4,41,61,63,67,70,77
Points (mortgage)	59
Power of Attorney	32
Prenuptial agreement	22
Probate	31,48,79,80
Profit sharing	30

F

Property	59,60,63-4
Puts, investment	66
Ratings, investments & insurance	41,68
Real estate	44
Record keeping (patient)	53,69
Rent	60,64-5
Rental property	43
Salary	19,25,33-4,55,67,81
Savings	9,37,41,46,71-2
Securities	7,39,43,51,54,59,61-5
SEC	73
Shareholder	27,33-4,62
SIPC	71
Solo practice	26
Standard and Poor's	68
Startup, practice	17,35
Statute of Limitations	54
Stock	27,40,45,57,62,72-3
Stock broker	8,56
Sublet	64
Suits, legal	27,34,49,54
Tax-deferred	5
Tax-exempt	61
Taxes	3,4,13,14,18,22,28,31,36, 67,69,73,75,80-1

G

Testator	80
Trust	6,28,44,75
Trustee	80
U.S. Gov't securities	46,50,72
Umbrella insurance	49
Vesting, pension	77
Vicarious liability	78
Will	32,48,74,79,80
Withholding tax	81
Workmen's compensation	24
Zero-coupon security	82

ORDER FORM

- ♦ Fax inquiries - (718) 278-0354
- ♦ Tel. inquiries - (718) 278-7676
  (800) 637-4644
- ♦ Mail orders:
  Baffin Books, Inc.
  4601 Broadway
  Astoria, NY 11103

Please send ____ copies of:

DOCTOR-TO-DOCTOR: AVOIDING FINANCIAL SUICIDE

to: _____
   _____
   _____

Payment: Prepaid $12.95 US in check or money order (no cash, credit cards, or COD's, please). Postage paid in USA. New York residents - add sales tax.

ORDER FORM

- ♦ Fax inquiries - (718) 278-0354
- ♦ Tel. inquiries -(718) 278-7676
  (800) 637-4644
- ♦ Mail orders:
  Baffin Books, Inc.
  4601 Broadway
  Astoria, NY 11103

Please send ____ copies of:

DOCTOR-TO-DOCTOR: AVOIDING FINANCIAL SUICIDE

to: _____
   _____
   _____

Payment: Prepaid $12.95 US in check or money order (no cash, credit cards, or COD's, please). Postage paid in USA. New York residents - add sales tax.